Medicare
Alphabet
Chaos

Lynn H. Zaffke

The goal of this book is to help you understand Medicare and retirement decisions.

Table of Contents

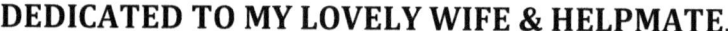

DEDICATED TO MY LOVELY WIFE & HELPMATE.

YOU QUALIFY FOR

MEDICARE PART A

BY

WORKING & PAYING

TAXES

CHAPTER 1

MEDICARE CONFUSION

HAS LEARNING ABOUT MEDICARE been difficult? Do you feel frustrated or overwhelmed by trying to choose a plan? Many people going on Medicare are in this situation. There are so many alphabet letters and acronyms that define the Medicare plans. It causes Medicare confusion.

Medicare is NOT like the insurance policy that you had during your working career. Medical insurance obtained through work provides a few plans. Companies offer about three insurance plans making the decision process almost painless. The government and private insurance companies offer numerous Medicare options producing confusion.

Overview

You may have heard of the term Original Medicare. It is Medicare Part A and Medicare Part B insurance policies offered by the government. Medicare Part A is for hospital coverage, and Part B covers outpatient services.

Part A and Part B will not cover all your medical expenses.

Medicare Part C is a synonym for Medicare Advantage. An Advantage plan will manage your health care. Private insurance companies offer them and are reimbursed by Medicare. Medicare A and B are administered by the insurance company so they can no longer be called Original. Someone enrolled in a Medicare Advantage Plan has given his/her rights for Original Medicare to their insurance company for management of their health care.

Supplement plans may be purchased separately from Original Medicare. Private insurance companies provide these. Supplement plans will pay whatever Medicare doesn't pay within certain limits. These plans have alphabet names. There are plans A, B, C, D, E, F, HDF, G, K, L, M, and N.

Medicare Part D is a drug plan that may be purchased to pay for prescription medicines.

The annual enrollment period is from October 15th through December 7th. Plans begin on January 1st of the next year.

What you will need for the best insurance coverage is Medicare A and B, a drug plan and either an Advantage or Supplement Plan. Let's expand these areas of Medicare.

CHAPTER 2

MEDICARE PART A

MEDICARE PART A IS HOSPITAL insurance coverage for qualified people over 65 years old. Part A is free health insurance offered by the government. To be eligible, you must work 40 quarters of time (or ten years). You may also be entitled to Medicare Part A because of your spouse's work history. If you haven't worked, but still want Medicare coverage, you can pay a premium to get it. Apply for Medicare about three months before your 65th birthday.

Medicare Part A covers hospitalization costs. It has a per-occurrence deductible which can vary from year to year. If you have hospital admissions more than 60 days apart, there will be two deductible bills within that year.

Under certain conditions, skilled nursing care is covered by Medicare part A. This means it will pay for rehabilitation or nursing home care after hospitalization. The key to this reimbursement is rehabilitation. A person must participate in therapy and show improvement with a goal of discharge to home. It will not cover a long-term care illness. Individuals in rehab are regularly evaluated to determine if it is a temporary rehabilitation condition (getting better) or if it has become a long-term care situation.

Hospice is covered by Medicare A. Hospice is for end-of-life care during an illness with the expectation of imminent death. Coverage is for the final six months of life. It may include in-home assistance or a stay in a hospice facility.

Original Medicare doesn't pay for all medical bills. You must buy Medicare B for outpatient cost coverage.

Recap:

Medicare A Covers:

> Hospital Costs
>
> Skilled Nursing Care
>
> Hospice

Apply for Medicare 3 months before your 65th birthday.

CHAPTER 3

MEDICARE PART B

DURING YOUR WORKING CAREER, you paid for Medicare Part A, but not for Part B. This is the reason you pay a premium for Medicare Part B. Original Medicare (Part A) doesn't pay for all medical bills.

Medicare Part B covers outpatient care delivered in the clinic or an emergency room. It includes provider visits, tests, and same-day surgeries. It also includes blood work, X-rays, MRI's, CT scans, and ambulance.

Medicare Part B has a monthly premium which is charged based on your income. The amount of revenue is calculated by combining all sources of money coming to you in retirement. If your income reaches over $85,000.00 per year for a single person or $170,000.00 for a married couple, expect to pay a high premium. The cost is deducted directly out of your Social Security check.

The annual deductible amount and the Medicare Part B premiums are set by Congress and can vary in cost from year to year. The 2017 Medicare Part B annual deductible price is $183.00. Once the deductible price

YOU MUST PAY

FOR

MEDICARE PART B

of $183.00 has been paid, Medicare Part B becomes an 80/20 percent plan. You are responsible for the deductible ($183.00) plus 20 percent of the bill. This 20 percent can quickly add up to a significant out-of-pocket bill. There is no limit with original Medicare Part B for out-of-pocket expenses.

You may see something called Excess Doctor Charges. Hospitals and providers can charge 15 percent more than Medicare will agree to pay. The patient will be responsible for the additional 15 percent.

Excess Doctor Charges are becoming more prevalent because of the government squeeze put upon providers. Private hospitals/providers may be more inclined to charge these fees.

Recap: Medicare Part B

Medicare Part B covers outpatient care delivered in the clinic or an emergency room.

You must pay a premium for Medicare Part B.

Once the deductible price has been met, Medicare Part B becomes an 80/20 percent plan.

PART C
IS
MANAGED CARE

CHAPTER 4

MEDICARE PART C: ADVANTAGE PLAN

MEDICARE ADVANTAGE PLAN is synonymous with Medicare Part C. It is a managed health care plan, like a Health Maintenance Organization (HMO) or a Preferred Provider Organization (PPO). The insurance company administers the customer's health plan and access to providers. When you enroll in such a plan, you agree to have your medical decisions to be managed by the insurance company.

In the Medicare Advantage Plan system, all medical treatments must be approved by the insurance company. Prior authorizations for surgery and procedures are necessary.

Advantage plans usually come with a prescription drug plan, vision plan, hearing aid allowance, and limited dental coverage. These even require prior authorization.

To receive healthcare, you must choose from the provider network. A provider is defined as a physician, physician assistant or a nurse practitioner. Using a network sets limits for your choice of providers. You may have to give up your current provider unless of course, he/she happens to be in the network. Measure your willingness to change practitioners.

MEDICARE ADVANTAGE

IS

ANOTHER NAME

FOR

MEDICARE PART C

Providers may opt out of a network any time during the year. This opt-in/opt-out system creates a changing network of providers.

Healthy people have the easiest time changing providers. If a consistent provider is not necessarily important to you, then an Advantage Plan may be a good choice. If you have chronic health issues, (diabetes, heart problems, or cancer,) changing providers can be frustrating or even dangerous. Handling these health problems is better with some continuity of care.

The advantage of Medicare Advantage Plans is that they have low premiums. Some Advantage Plans even have a zero premium. But, don't be fooled, Advantage Plans are not free. Charges include copays and coinsurance for services. For example, to have a provider appointment, the insurance company pays most of the bill, except the pre-determined copay of $15.00. The copay is a pre-established amount for this service.

Coinsurance may be charged for a procedure. Coinsurance is an 80/20 percent coverage. The insurance company is accountable for 80 percent of the bill. The client is responsible for 20 percent. The actual amount of the bill will be calculated using the two methods of copay and coinsurance until the out of pocket limit is reached.

A shortcoming of a Medicare Advantage Plan is that plans are not constant from year to year. The networks and prices can change, and the plans can even be discontinued. Once a plan is withdrawn, you must find a new Medicare Advantage Plan.

Buying a Medicare Advantage Plan is a gamble. You will be gambling that you will stay healthy. If you are diagnosed with a major health issue, the costs of health care could be devastating.

Medicare Advantage Plans are restricted by geography. There are plans available everywhere, but the plans are limited by region. They may only be available in certain counties, or even certain Zip Codes in a state. If you buy a plan in Florida but later, relocate to Georgia, you must enroll in a new plan. There is a special enrollment period for your new location. This period begins the month before you move. It lasts four months. For example, let us say you relocate in May. The special enrollment period begins the first of April; it will include May, June, and July.

Most Medicare Advantage Plans have an agreement with network doctors, so they do not charge Excess Doctor Charges to the patients.

MEDICAID/MEDICARE PART C

There are unique Medicare Part C Plans available for people on Medicaid/Medicare. These are called Dual Eligible Plans. These are usually free, and there is no co-pay. The value of the Medicaid/Medicare plan is that the Medicaid will oversee your medical care.

The Dual Eligible Plan will require you to choose a provider in the network. The plan will pay for all provider appointments and all medications.

Primarily, the Dual Eligible Plan helps you manage your health care problems. Many services are available to manage chronic diseases. Benefits may include in-home nursing wellness visits. Usually, there is a 24/7 nurse hotline. For example, if you have diabetes, a diabetic care plan will provide assistance to monitor your blood glucose levels to help determine the amount of insulin or oral medication needed.

Recap: Medicare Part C

Medicare Part C is synonymous to a Medicare Advantage Plan.

Advantage plans usually come with a prescription drug plan, vision plan, hearing aid allowance, and limited dental coverage.

Your provider must be in the network, and you may not be able to keep the same doctor year to year.

Advantage Plans are inexpensive.

Buying a Medicare Advantage Plan is gambling that you will stay healthy.

SUPPLEMENT PLANS

ARE

MEDIGAP PLANS

CHAPTER 5

MEDICARE SUPPLEMENT PLANS

MEDICARE SUPPLEMENT PLANS are entirely different from Medicare Advantage plans. A Medicare Supplement Plan has a premium paid to the insurance company. You keep your Medicare rights. When Medicare approves a cost, it must be paid by the insurance company. If a provider accepts Medicare, they will take this plan. There are no networks within a supplement plan.

Medicare Supplement plans are referred to as Medigap plans. There are plans A, B, C, D, F, HDF, G, K, L, M, and N. Some of these plans may not be available in your state.

The Center for Medicare & Medicaid Services (CMS) standardizes all Medicare Supplement plans to ensure all insurance plans are the same from one company to the next. All the businesses that offer Plan F must adhere to the framework set by CMS. In other words, all F Plans are the same thing.

The difference from company to company is the cost of the monthly or annual premiums you pay. The cost variance can be quite large! The charge may be up to $100.00 per month more between the least expensive plan to the most expensive plan. You do NOT get what you pay for since there are no differences in the benefits that the plans will provide.

Supplement plans have guaranteed benefits. If the premium is paid, the benefits cannot change year to year.

What are the benefits of supplement plans? Let's use Plan G as an example. After receiving care, the customer pays the annual Medicare Part B deductible. Once the deductible is met, all other Medicare approved charges are paid 100%.

Supplement plans have a premium that needs to be paid by the customer. Plan F has the highest premium, meaning it is the most expensive. It has the best coverage making it the most attractive. All medical bills will have 100 percent coverage paid either by Medicare or the Supplement Plan F insurance company.

 The next most comprehensive plan is Plan G. The monthly premiums for Plan F and G are about the same. Plan N is also purchased often.

Notably, Medicare Plan F, Plan C, and the high-deductible Plan F will be discontinued in 2020. For this reason, you may want to avoid these three plans. Plan F will remain in place for those people who have purchased it before 2020. Historically the premiums for a discontinued plan have increased in the years following. Increases have been as high as 15 percent. If you are looking for a bargain, these plans are poor choices. New plans will not be introduced in 2020.

No Medicare Supplement Plan has a drug plan included. It is up to you to enroll in a stand-alone drug plan to cover prescription drug costs.

It is important to know which companies have a good track record with their customers. Some companies are rated higher than others because of their business practices. An "A" rating for a company is based on their finances, but not their customer service. Do not depend on the ratings to help you choose the plan.

An agent will suggest plans from multiple companies. He/she is most likely to have your best interests in mind. An agent will know the companies with good customer service ratings and good pricing.

The best time to get a Medicare Supplement Plan is at age 65 when you are hopefully still healthy. You may be required to qualify for a supplement plan. If you wait until an older age, it may be more problematic to meet the health requirements. The average senior has health problems in their 70-80's. If you fall into the average senior category, waiting to purchase a plan will be a costly decision. It is not impossible to get a plan at an older age, but it could be frustrating and expensive.

If you choose not to get a plan, you will pay for the deductible for Part A and Part B, the 20 percent of Part B that is not covered by Medicare and there will be unlimited liability for your portion of the 20 percent.

SUPPLEMENT PLANS

HAVE

GUARANTEED BENEFITS

BUT

YOU PAY FOR IT

Recap:

There are no Networks with a supplement plan.

There will be no difference in a plan from one company to the next.

Do not depend on the company ratings to help you choose the plan.

The best time to get a Medicare Supplement Plan is at age 65 when you are still healthy.

Supplement Plans have guaranteed benefits but have a premium that must be paid by the customer.

What is the difference between a Medicare Advantage Plan and a Medicare Supplement Plan?

Chart A

	Benefits	**Network**
Medicare Advantage Plan	Changes year to year	You must be in a network. Networks have opt-in/out and providers may change
Medicare Supplement Plan	Guaranteed, does not change	No Network. No referrals needed. You choose your own provider

Chart A continued...

	Drug Plan	Pre- approval
Medicare Advantage Plan	Your Drug Plan is usually included in the plan	You need pre-approval from insurance for procedures and/or medical treatments
Medicare Supplement Plan	You must buy a stand-alone drug plan	Procccd with medical procedures as needed or guided by your MD

SUPPLEMENT PLANS

ARE THE

SAME

NO MATTER WHICH COMPANY

YOU CHOOSE

CHAPTER 6

HOW TO CHOOSE A MEDICARE SUPPLEMENT PLAN IN 30 MINUTES OR LESS.

PEOPLE OF THE TURNING 65 group get bombarded by mail and phone calls regarding Medicare Health Plans. Instead of educating the recipient, it causes confusion. Reading every company's material muddies the information. Each insurance company puts their spin on the plans because, of course, they are pitching their business.

Recall the discussion that Medicare Supplement plans are standardized by the government. These plans are designed to pay the additional health care costs that are not covered by Original Medicare. These expenses include deductibles, copayments, and coinsurance. All plans are the same no matter which company you choose.

It is not necessary to decide your plan or what is best for you before a consulting meeting with an agent. Identifying the desired plan before a meeting will streamline the consulting time. Assess your health needs. Assess your pocketbook.

Let's make it simple. Take fifteen minutes and read about five pages in the Medicare and You 2017 Handbook.

This booklet was mailed to you by Medicare. If you don't have one, you can find it online at www.medicare.gov. The Supplement information is in Section 6, pages 81 to 84.

The chart on page 82 of the 2017 Medicare and You Handbook displays coverage for each Medicare Supplement Plan. (See Chart B.) Benefits are identical for all the plans in Medicare Part A and cover 100 percent of hospitalization. All plans (except Plans K and L) cover Medicare Part B co-insurance, the first three units of blood, and Hospice Care. The bottom part of the chart is where the differences in the plans are noted.

Again, all plans are standardized to be the same from company to company. Choosing a Plan C will be the same plan no matter which company offers it. The plan differences are the name of the company and of course, the price. The monthly costs may vary quite a bit.

The next step is to look at one company's informational material. That's right, just look at one company's information. It will explain the plans simply. It is not necessary to buy your plan from this company, but their material will be duplicated by every other business. All the plans are the same due to government regulation.

Recap: How to choose a Medicare Supplement Plan in 30 minutes or less.

Read about five pages in the Medicare and You 2017 Handbook.

Look at one company's material to learn each plan.

Meet with a qualified insurance agent to purchase your plan.

The following chart has been adapted from:

Medicare Supplement (Medigap) Plans Chart B

https://www.medicare.gov/pubs/pdf/10050.pdf,pg.82

	A	B	C	D	F
Medicare A Coinsurances & Hospital	100%	100%	100%	100%	100%
Medicare Part B Coinsurance	100%	100%	100%	100%	100%
Blood-3 pints	100%	100%	100%	100%	100%
Part A Hospice	100%	100%	100%	100%	100%
Skilled Nursing			100%	100%	100%
Part A Deductible		100%	100%	100%	100%
Part B Deductible			100%		100%
Part B Excess Charge					100%
Foreign-Travel (up to plan limits)			80%	80%	80%

	G	K	L	M	N
Medicare A Coinsurances & Hospital	100%	100%	100%	100%	100%
Medicare Part B Coinsurance	100%	50%	75%	100%	100% $20 copay
Blood-3 pints	100%	50%	75%	100%	100%
Part A Hospice	100%	50%	75%	100%	100%
Skilled Nursing	100%	50%	75%	100%	100%
Part A Deductible	100%	50%	75%	100%	100%
Part B Deductible					
Part B Excess Charge	100%				
Foreign Travel	80%	Out of Pocket limit $4960	Out of pocket limit $2480	80%	80%

MEDICARE PART D IS AN OPTIONAL DRUG PLAN

CHAPTER 7

MEDICARE PART D (OPTIONAL PRESCRIPTION DRUG PLAN)

THE STANDARD FRAMEWORK of a Prescription Drug Plan is set by CMS. The insurance companies can add to that foundation, but they cannot go below this threshold. Consequently, drug plans are very similar from one insurance company to the next. The differences include the formularies, co-pay differences, and coinsurance for the drugs.

A drug plan has a formulary which is a list of medicines that would be covered by the drug plan. A prescription drug plan can and will change every year. When a drug becomes available as a generic drug, the insurance company can drop the name-brand drug from their formulary and replace it with the generic drug version.

The formularies have tiered levels. Tier 1 and 2 are usually generic drugs. Name-brand drugs and specialty drugs are tiered in 3-5 levels. The upper tiers have higher copays or coinsurance connected with the prescription.

A co-pay is a set amount such as $25.00. Coinsurance, on the other hand, is a percentage of the cost of the drug.

For example, 33 percent may be the required percentage of coinsurance that you would pay for medicine.

Most drug plans have a deductible amount which must be paid before the copays or coinsurance begins. Some plans, (especially mail order) will not charge for generic level 1 or 2 drugs.

If you only take generic prescription drugs, look for a plan with no deductible. Or, check for a plan that does not charge for generic tier 1 or tier 2 drugs. It will save you money.

It is imperative to review your drug plan every fall during the annual enrollment period. The formularies may vary, pharmacies change, and the type of medication needed may change. During annual enrollment, you can change your drug or Medicare Advantage plan without a penalty. It will not be necessary to give a health history.

Call the Medicare hotline (1-800-Medicare), and they will help you find the least expensive drug plan for you. Some insurance agents provide this service for their clients.

Occasionally, retirement programs offer health insurance and a prescription drug insurance. Check with the Human Resource department from your former employer to see if this is your case. You cannot have a Part D plan and keep the retirement coverage. It may impact your spouse if your plan covers your dependents.

Drugs administered in the emergency room will be paid by the prescription drug plan. This adds to the drug costs and may drive a patient to go into the donut hole.

If admitted to the hospital, the medicines administered will be an expense for Medicare Part A.

The government prefers for people get a drug plan when they turn 65 years old. If you wait to enroll, there is a late enrollment penalty. It is the government's way of encouraging you to get a prescription drug plan at age 65 and not wait until later. Getting a prescription drug plan after age 65 forces you to pay a higher premium. It is a cumulative penalty which never goes away.

Recap:

The differences in drug plans include the formularies, co-pay differences, and coinsurance for the drugs.

Most drug plans have a deductible amount which must be paid before the copays or coinsurance begins.

Waiting to buy a drug plan after age 65 will force you to pay a huge penalty in premiums.

Call 1-800-Medicare to find an appropriate drug plan, or ask your insurance agent to assist you.

THE DONUT HOLE
IS THE
DRUG
COVERAGE GAP

CHAPTER 8

WHAT IS THE DONUT HOLE?

THE DONUT HOLE IS THE COVERAGE gap that starts when drug costs reach a set amount. The amount for 2017 is $3700.00. Depending on your plan, you may have up to a $400.00 deductible. In the initial coverage phase you pay a share of the cost of your drugs and Medicare Part D picks up the rest.

Once you reach the set limit ($3700.00) of real drug costs, you reach the Donut Hole. This is calculated using the actual cost of the medicine. For example, if you pay a $20.00 copayment for a $100.00 drug, the retail value of the drug is $100.00. This retail value counts as the actual cost toward the limit.

Once you have met that maximum dollar amount, you are officially in the donut hole. You are responsible for the rest of your drug bills for the remainder of the year or until you have reached the catastrophic coverage level. The coverage gap is calculated from the beginning of each calendar year. This amount includes out-of-pocket and plan-paid dollars. Basically, if you pay more than $308.00 dollars per month for your medicines, you will hit the donut hole.

HOW DO I GET OUT OF THE DONUT HOLE?

In 2017, the magic get out of the donut hole number is $4850.00 of paid out-of-pocket expenses. This number gets you out of the donut hole/coverage gap and changes your status to catastrophic coverage. When you reach catastrophic coverage, you pay either a five percent coinsurance for covered drugs or a copay of $2.95 for covered generic drugs and $7.40 for covered brand-name drugs, whichever is greater.

You must continue to pay the monthly premium during your coverage gap. Your premium does not count toward the $4,850.00 out-of-pocket limit. The amount your drug plan paid for your drugs in your initial coverage period also does not count toward the donut hole number. Only the money you contributed counts toward your $4,850.00 out of pocket expense.

The Medicare drug plan will total the out-of-pocket dollars on your covered prescription drugs during the year. The monthly Medicare statement will list this information.

Recap:

The donut hole is the drug coverage gap.

Paying $4,850.00 out-of-pocket expenses changes your status to catastrophic coverage.

CHAPTER 9

THE BEST ADVICE IN THE BOOK

SELECT A REPUTABLE, informed insurance broker who represents several companies to ensure finding a reasonable premium. Ask if he/she is a captured agent representing just one company. Find an agent that represents more than one company.

A good agent is an asset. He/she will review your personal situation and assist in choosing a plan that meets your needs. The agent can look over many companies and get the most affordable, appropriate Medicare plan. Compare an insurance agent to a lawyer or a physician. He/she will assess or diagnose your needs and recommend the correct plan for you. The agent is licensed and is an expert. Take advantage of this expertise. A good agent will save you money. In fact, a good agent can even make you money.

Essentially, the consult is free. The agent gets paid by the company. You do not pay anything for this expert advice. The agent can review your Social Security benefits as well. They know many ways to save money that the average person would not anticipate.

Many people contact the insurance company and buy their plan without an agent. Do it yourself insurance buying is not wise. Think about the phrase 'only fools represent themselves in court.' Buying insurance directly from the company is like representing yourself in court.

An agent having access to multiple companies will connect you with the correct plan for your situation. The agent will be able to keep your budget and needs in mind to choose the right Medicare Plan. Remember, this comes at no personal cost to you. In fact, it will likely save you a lot of money in the long term.

For example, a person with diabetes chooses a Medicare Advantage Plan. Diabetes is an expensive disease. A more appropriate Medicare Plan is a Medicare Supplement Plan. These plans have better coverage and less money out of pocket.

Take, for example, the couple that did their calculations for Social Security. They were skeptical that an agent could help them, but they met with the agent anyway. After the analysis, they found they were eligible for an extra $9,600.00 in Social Security benefits per year. The extra money started the next month. Predict these increases of income out for their average lifetime. They made an extra $250,000.00. Is this beneficial to them? They think so!

It doesn't work that way for everyone, but typically after a professional analysis, you will know that you have gained the best possible benefit from your Social Security.

You deserve the most from your Medicare and Social Security benefits because you faithfully paid those taxes your whole working life. It is the promise that the government has made to you as a retiree. Make certain to get the entire benefit.

Recap: The Best Advice in the Book.

Use an expert agent.

Having an agent will save you money in Medicare insurance plans and Social Security.

SPECIAL HELP
IS AVAILABLE
FOR
PEOPLE
WITH
LOW INCOME

CHAPTER 10

MEDICARE EXTRA HELP

MEDICARE EXTRA HELP is a federal program that assists you for payment of prescription drugs. It is available from Social Security, designed to help people on the lower income tiers.

Eligibility for Extra Help is calculated based on your total income from all retirement accounts. Singles making $1,505.00 or couples making $2,022.00 per month with assets below specific limits may be eligible for Extra Help. These income levels change every year.

Check if you are eligible for Medicare Extra Help. Go to www.ssa.gov and put Extra Help in the search bar and follow the instructions. Often, the Extra Help is on a sliding scale. The Extra Help program is designed to help pay for the cost of your drugs and may even pay the premium for your prescription drug plan.

Receiving Extra Help creates year-round open enrollment for a drug plan. Getting Extra Help allows a person to change plans during the year without taking a health history. Qualifying for Extra Help will nullify any late enrollment penalty that may be in effect. Be sure to check it out every year.

People enrolled in Medicare Savings Program (MSP), Supplemental Security Income (SSI) or Medicaid will automatically be qualified for Medicare Extra Help. However, you must fill out an application through the Social Security.

If you don't qualify for Medicaid, you may still qualify for Social Security Extra Help. There is a full or partial Extra Help plan. Your income and assets will determine the plan you will receive.

Get a private plan offering Medicare Drug coverage, even if you qualify for Medicare Extra Help. The plan must be in your geographical area. This plan will cover the necessary costs and must have a premium at or below the Extra Help premium amount for your state. A prescription drug plan is not mandatory. If you are not on any prescription drugs or you are taking a few generic drugs, you do not have to get a drug plan.

Once enrolled in Extra Help, you won't have to pay the full cost of your drugs. You must, of course, take the medications that are on your plan's formulary. Additionally, there is a requirement to purchase the medicines at a pharmacy in the plan's network.

Mail order prescriptions have certain rules and advantages. In some cases, for the same cost of a one-month supply of medicine, you may be allowed to get a 90-day supply.

If you qualify for Extra Help with your drug plan, the late enrollment penalty is waived.

Recap:

Medicare Extra Help is a federal program that assists low income people for payment of prescription drugs.

Receiving Extra Help creates year-round open enrollment for a drug plan or Medicare Advantage Prescription Drug Plan.

Extra Help is complicated with separate rules for qualifications and assets, but it is worth checking it out on the government website.

SOCIAL SECURITY

&

MEDICARE

ARE

SEPARATE PROGRAMS

CHAPTER 11

SOCIAL SECURITY

SOCIAL SECURITY AND MEDICARE are two different government programs. Even informed people are confused about them being a combined program. Due to this misperception, people make the decision to begin their Social Security at the same time they become eligible for Medicare. You do not have to take Social Security just because you become qualified for Medicare.

Social Security pays you a monthly check from the time you take it until you pass away. You have a choice of the timing of starting your Social Security payments.

It is important to take Social Security at the right time and the right way. If you take your Social Security before your full retirement age, be prepared for consequences of less retirement income. If you decide to continue to work, there is a limit to how much money you can make. If you make too much money, the Social Security department will reduce your Social Security check. (Isn't it hard to believe that someone can make too much money?)

At age 66, which is full retirement age, income is no longer limited. After full retirement age, Social Security benefits are not affected by how much other income you may make.

The Social Security office personnel cannot give advice. Do not go to an appointment at the Social Security office expecting assistance for decision making. Indeed, many Social Security employees do not understand the ramifications that occur when people take their social security at the wrong time. A mistaken decision can cost you thousands of dollars every year over the course of your retirement. It can mean the difference between having enough money during retirement or constantly having to economize.

Ask your insurance agent to run an analysis on Social Security. Agents should do this for clients at no charge. An analysis will be a beneficial tool for decision making for taking Social Security the right way and at the precise time.

Once you start your Social Security benefits you are not necessarily locked in at that position for your lifetime; rather you may make limited changes in your benefits up to the age of 70 years old within that year.

Too many people depend solely on their Social Security monies for retirement. Therefore, it is important to get as much money from Social Security as possible. Think about the significance of increasing the Social Security monthly income by just $100.00 more per month. Multiply $100.00 by twelve months, and you will have made $1200.00 more in one year.

Perhaps you will collect benefits for 20 years, which equals $24,000.00 more in retirement income. What could you do with some extra money?

The income benefit amounts paid from Social Security may increase from year to year. These increases are not indexed to inflation which is very unfair to seniors.

The Cost of Living Adjustment (COLA) is how Social Security adjusts your benefits to the government's definition of inflation.   For instance, the real inflation for 2017 is about 3 percent, but the COLA was 0.3 percent. This did not cover the increase in the Medicare Part B premium. Here are the COLA's for the last nine years.

2008: 5.8%	2013: 1.5%
2009: 0.0%	2014: 1.7%
2010: 0.0%	2015: 0.0%
2011: 3.6%	2016: 0.3%
2012: 1.7%	2017: 0.3%

Recap:

Take Social Security at the right time.

Social Security personnel cannot give advice.

Get a free Social Security analysis.

A GOOD AGENT

WILL

SAVE YOU

MONEY

CHAPTER 12

SOCIAL SECURITY: TAKE IT EARLY

MANY PEOPLE DESIRE to take their Social Security checks as soon as possible, at 62 years old. What they may not count on is their longevity. Americans are living longer than ever before. According to the US government, "The typical 65-year-old will live to age 83, One in four 65-year-olds will live to age 90, and one in ten 65-year-olds will live to age 95."

According to the U.S. Census Bureau, "Once we reach age 65, we can expect to live 17 more years. During the 1980's, post-65 life expectancy improved for all race/sex groups."

Taking Social Security early limits your income for the rest of your life. There are only two good reasons for taking your Social Security check early.

The first reason is that you have plenty of money in other retirement savings accounts making your Social Security check a less important source of income. Secondly, if you have a health issue and need to stop working then taking Social Security at age 62 may be a good option. However, if your health is at risk, you could explore the possibility of qualifying for disability instead. Once you are on disability, you will be paid your full retirement amount.

Search life expectancy, on the internet for a person with your disease or ailment. Getting the facts about life expectancy can empower your decision making. If you think your life will be shortened, take Social Security early.

When you retire at age 62, your check could hypothetically, be about $1200.00 per month. The check amount depends, of course, on how much money you made during your working years. The money becomes a frozen value plus the cost of living allowance.

For example, Janis was told by her friends to take her Social Security right away at 62 years old. "You never know if you'll die young... so take the money while you can!" Without consulting a qualified agent, Janis chose to take her Social Security money, yet continued to work.

Since she took her Social Security at the age of 62, there was a limit for how much money she could earn. Her total benefits for the rest of her life were affected because she heeded the unprofessional advice of well-meaning friends and took her social security too early. Her retirement income was drastically reduced.

Many friends who give us free advice do not understand the filing options for Social Security and their consequences. People make the mistake of filing at the wrong time and thus affecting not only their retirement income but also their spouse's retirement income.

Make sure to maximize your benefits. Social Security will pay you for the rest of your life and the rest of your spouse's life.   Don't shortchange yourselves by making the wrong choice.

Yearly statements are available from the Social Security Administration. Sometimes they send the statement by U.S. Mail. You can view your statement online. You must create a Social Security account. Find it at: www.socialsecurity.gov/myaccount.

This report gives you your earnings history and the amount of taxes you and/or your employer has paid toward Social Security and Medicare. You will find out your estimated payment if you retire at the full retirement age making approximately the same amount of money at present. The statement gives estimated benefits for retirement, disability, and family survivors.

Recap:

If you take Social Security at age 62, you will have less money than if you would have waited.

Check out your personalized Social Security account.

YOU MAKE MORE MONEY WHEN YOU TAKE SOCIAL SECURITY LATER

CHAPTER 13

SOCIAL SECURITY TIMING: TAKE IT LATER

WE WORK HARD and look forward to retirement. Relaxation, trips, family times, grandchildren and learning new things may be in the future. If you retire early and run out of money, retirement won't be much fun. You need to plan for retirement and a long life. Let's look at why waiting for Social Security benefits might be wise.

Statistically, both men and women in good health at age 65 can expect to live to be 87-89 years old. This means delaying Social Security benefits until full retirement age (66) or later will provide a healthy person much more money in retirement.

Delaying Social Security benefits until an older age increases the amount of the check for every postponed year. Waiting until your full retirement age will significantly increase the Social Security check. If you can wait until age 70, your Social Security check will be at its highest peak. In fact, waiting until age 70 may more than double the amount of money when compared to taking benefits at age 62 years old.

 Your Social Security benefits will grow approximately

8 percent per year. At age 70 you are required take Social Security.

About 90 percent of people retiring have less than $20,000.00 in savings. If this is you, and you depend on Social Security as your primary source of income, then a good strategy for timing is vital. If this is your plan, be smart. Wait to retire and postpone taking your Social Security.

At age 62, the average American will make $12,000.00 per year.

If deferred to age 70, that money will grow about 8 percent per year to about $21,000.00 per year.

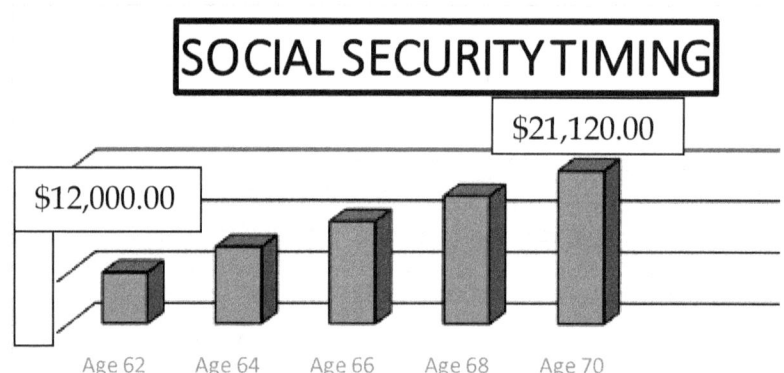

SOCIAL SECURITY TIMING

$21,120.00

$12,000.00

Age 62   Age 64   Age 66   Age 68   Age 70

Your social security check will increase by about 8 percent per year for every year delayed. For instance, were let's say you were to get $1,000.00 per month at your full retirement age of 66. If you waited until you were 67, you would get another $80.00 per month. Multiply that by 12 months that would be an extra $960.00 per year. It doesn't sound like much in one year, but if you multiply it by a possible 25 years of living until 85 or 90 years old, an extra $960.00 per year would be mean another $25,000.00 in your retirement. It adds up.

Delaying Social Security until age 70 will increase your social security check by 32 percent higher than if you took it at full retirement age of 66 years old.

Here is another example. Joan is in excellent health. Her parents, aunts, and uncles lived into their 90's. At her full retirement age of 66, her Social Security benefit is $1,500.00 per month. If she waited until age 70 to take Social Security, she would have a monthly benefit increase by $480.00 more per month. It is $1,980.00 per month or $5,760.00 more per year. If she lives to age 90, she will receive an additional $115,200.00 in her retirement.

You may be wondering about the money Joan didn't take from age 66 to age 70. It adds up to about $72,000.00. Subtract the $72,000.00 from $115,200.00. This is equal to $43,200.00 that she would have gained. Joan is ahead $43,200.00 by waiting four years to collect benefits. If she chose to work those years and have a salary, she will have gained even more income.

The break-even point of delaying your Social Security until age 70 by a single person is about 79 years old. The average healthy woman will live about 24 years past retirement. To ensure money throughout those 24 or so years, delaying taking your Social Security and working longer substantially increases your retirement finances.

Recap: Take Social Security at the right time and the right way.

Medicare and Social Security are two separate programs. You do not need to take Social Security when you sign up for Medicare.

Age 66, is full retirement age. After this, Social Security benefits are not affected by how much other income you may make.

Get a Social Security analysis before making decisions.

You may make limited changes in your benefits up to the age of 70 years old.

CHAPTER 14

SPOUSAL BENEFITS

MODIFICATION OF SPOUSAL BENEFITS occurred in the last year. Congress enacted new laws that changed the file and suspend strategy.

File and suspend can still be done at the older age and it is a good tactic for healthy couples. The spouse with the largest income should postpone his/her retirement benefit and wait until age 70 to collect the Social Security benefit at the top value. A couple will make much more money letting the larger of the two Social Security benefits grow.

The strategy looks like this. It consists of one spouse taking their Social Security benefit. Pick the smaller of the two Social Security checks while the larger one continues to grow. The other spouse applies for the spousal benefit. A couple collects one complete check and half of the same full check for the other spouse.

For example, a wife can take her benefit, say $1,200.00 a month. Her husband can take the spousal benefit of $600.00 a month. This will allow the husband's Social Security benefits to continue to grow at about 8 percent per year until he would reach age 70. At that time, he would relinquish the spousal benefit and be required to take his own Social Security benefits.

The benefits will be much more per month because of the 8 percent growth per year. This strategy is an excellent way to maximize your Social Security benefits and perhaps relieve some financial stress in retirement.

Spousal benefits must be calculated on a per couple basis as there are many variations.

Re-cap:

Using the Spousal Benefit strategy, a couple can get 1 ½ times the amount of the lower Social Security check. You can still collect money while letting one Social Security account grow by 8 percent per year until the age of 70 years old.

CHAPTER 15

STRATEGIES FOR DIVORCED PERSONS

SOME DIVORCED PEOPLE are qualified for Spousal Benefits. A person married 10 or more years to the same person can apply for this benefit. You qualify for this if you did not remarry.

Spousal Benefit acknowledges that during the married years, you were helping your ex-spouse. Whether this was for managing the home or working outside the home makes no difference. A divorced person can be eligible for up to one-half of the social security check from the ex-spouse. The money does not come out of the Social Security check belonging to the ex-spouse. It is a separate government adjustment. If you take the spousal benefit, you can let your benefits grow.

Using this strategy may enable the divorced person to be eligible for extra thousands of dollars per year. Divorced spouses can even claim their ex-spouse's total social security check upon his/her death.

For divorced persons that fit the Spousal Benefit of the Social Security's criteria, the best time and strategy to take your benefits is after full retirement age.

SPOUSAL BENEFITS
MAY NET YOU
MORE MONEY

CHAPTER 16

UNMARRIED COUPLES-LIVING TOGETHER

COUPLES LIVING TOGETHER but not legally married should try to maximize Social Security benefits. File as a single.

If you marry, your finances merge, but when living together they do not. Think ahead of what happens when one of you dies. Discuss the finances. Realize that you are in a partnership. Have a will or legal document that anticipates the death of one in the partnership.

Plan for illness. Get a health care power of attorney so you can choose who makes your health care decisions. Plan how you will cover health care expenses. Get Long Term Care insurance. If one of you goes on Medicaid, the other will not be responsible for the bills unless you have joint accounts or assets.

Who will inherit your money upon death? If married, the spouse is the presumed heir. It doesn't work that way if you live together. No doubt you do not want your partner kicked to the curb by children who show up to the funeral. Plan. Decide your wishes together so there are no surprises upon death.

DID YOU SAVE ENOUGH MONEY FOR RETIREMENT?

CHAPTER 17

RETIREMENT ACCOUNTS

NOT ENOUGH PEOPLE take advantage of individual retirement accounts. Our saving rate as a country is abysmal. Saving money has not been the American priority. The incomes have not kept up to our lifestyles and cost of living. We all have plenty of places to spend money. It takes a high income and a lot of self-discipline to save for retirement.

When approaching retirement age, scrutinize your retirement accounts. Determine the type of lifestyle you will be able to have after retirement. Learn about the nuances of the accounts where your money is invested.

Retirement accounts, such as the 401k and 403b were developed in the late 1970's and early 1980's. Roth IRA's came later and were named after the Delaware Congressman William Roth who authored the bill. The 401k and 403b plans were named for the section of the tax code that governs them. These plans became popular because companies wanted to get out of the escalating costs of pension plans which were proving to be extremely expensive.

The retirement plans were designed to be an additional retirement income to be used in addition to Social

Security. The accounts were never intended to provide total retirement income. It was assumed Social Security would still be a primary source of revenue. Now, the opposite is true. According to the government, Social Security should make up only 40 percent of retirement income.

The 401k, 403b, IRA and Roth IRA accounts remain the primary retirement saving method for most people. Many employers sponsor these retirement plans as a benefit. In these plans, the companies may have matched the employee's contribution. All contributions to your 401k accounts are pre-tax money, meaning no taxes will be paid on your earnings during the year you earned it. You will owe taxes on it when you withdraw it during retirement. IRA accounts offer tax-deferred growth on investments, and like the 401k and 403b, these IRA accounts will not be taxed until money is withdrawn.

The Roth IRA is modeled after a life insurance policy without the benefits of life insurance. The tax was paid on income before making contributions to the Roth IRA. It makes retirement withdrawals tax free.

A Roth IRA may provide more spendable income in retirement. This account has a yearly limit on the money amount that can be saved. The Roth IRA can hold bonds, stocks, mutual funds, certificates of deposits and/or money market accounts within the account. These will be offered through banks and brokerage houses.

There are different tax advantages for a Roth IRA, but not everyone qualifies for a Roth IRA. The requirement is an adjusted gross income of less than $116,000.00, or $183,000.00 for married couples filing jointly.

The original strategy of the 401k, 403b, and traditional IRA was dependent on Social Security not being taxed. Withdrawals from these accounts is considered as income and therefore is taxable. In 1993 the government decided that Social Security would be included as income. Social Security benefits are now taxable at certain income levels.

You determine how your money is invested in a 401k or 403b plan. Most plans offer an array of mutual funds composed of stocks & bonds. There are plenty of restrictions and caveats with 401k and 403b accounts. There are complex rules about fund withdrawal and costly penalties if you take money out before retirement age.

IRA's, 401k and 403b accounts are often subject to stock market fluctuations. Losing money in your retirement accounts can be detrimental. It could cause you to run out of money quickly and force a personal financial disaster. Take the financial crisis of 2007-2008 as an example. People with stocks lost lots of money.

When or if the market goes down, a younger person has time to recover from the downturn. However, for an aging retiree with money invested in the stock market, a decline can empty or at least substantially reduce the account. Retirees do not have thirty or forty years to recover the lost stock market money. A retired person depends on this for living expenses and medical bills.

An annuity is an excellent option for retirement monies. However, annuities have gotten a bad reputation. The variable rate annuities are the villains. These annuities go up and down with the stock market and have many hidden fees. Do not transfer your money to a variable rate annuity.

Annuities have many different names and are offered by insurance agents and companies. Many types of safe annuities offer a lifetime payout. This payout gives you confidence that your income stream will continue to be payed to you until you die. If you have a lifetime payout, you will never run out of money. These annuities will guarantee payment even after the account has run out of money.

Some annuities offer a bonus upon transfer of your funds from another retirement account. The bonus makes it feel almost too good to be true. However, check into it. Most of the accounts are offered by reputable companies and have proven track records for good return in a safe, recession-proof account.

A fixed index annuity has a guaranteed rate of return. This has an emphasis on principle safety with a guaranteed interest rate. The insurance company provides predictable and stable investment returns.

Recap:

Analyze retirement accounts for withdrawal availability, risk, and tax consequences. Consider annuities or life insurance as a lower risk account.

CHAPTER 18

TAXES AND FINANCES

SOCIAL SECURITY WAS NON-TAXED income until 1993. The Congress and the President passed and signed a bill that made Social Security benefits taxable. In October 2015, the Congress passed the Omnibus Budget Bill. This was a bipartisan effort. This new tax literally has pickpocketed seniors of a staggering ten billion dollars a year.

The bill requires you to pay taxes on the money that your employer contributed to Social Security in your name.

The tax consequences of these congressional actions caused seniors to pay more taxes on other retirement monies. Changes also came in the Spousal Benefits.

The taxing of Social Security benefits could contribute to a cash shortage in retirement. Most people and some advisors neglect to include taxes in retirement analysis. Income projections should account for taxes. The pain of paying income tax increases when you have other significant income in your nest egg such as interest, dividends, self-employment, and wages.

Based on the rules from the Internal Revenue Service, you will pay income tax on up to 85 percent of your Social Security Benefits.

For example; at the 15 percent tax bracket, 85 percent of your Social Security check will be taxed at the rate of 15 percent.

If you work during retirement, as many people do, keep the income limits in mind. The more money earned increases the rate of the Social Security taxes. The extra income may not be worth the higher rate of taxation. Working may actually reduce your income. Talk to a tax accountant to learn your income limit for the next year.

The government has a program of Required Minimum Distribution (RMD) for IRA's and 401k's and 403b accounts. When you have reached age 70 ½, you are required to take money out of these accounts based on expected lifespan. The government demands the tax money. It is designed so the government will get the maximum amount of taxes from your accounts.

The government determines how much money you will be obligated to withdraw from your retirement accounts. This rule forces many seniors into a high tax bracket and prematurely empties these accounts. If you live "too long," you may run short of money because of these compulsory government mandated withdrawals. Money in Roth IRA and life insurance are exempt from this rule.

Some states have an income tax that piggybacks to federal income tax. For this reason, many retirees take advantage of moving to a state where there is no state income tax. Moving allows retirement money to last longer because they're not paying extra state taxes.

CHAPTER 19

LIFE EXPECTANCY

HOW LONG WILL YOU LIVE ONCE you have retired? That is the question we all ignore but should address. Why not be practical and estimate how long you could live? A life expectancy projection could assist you to plan your spending during the retirement years.

Here is what life expectancy looks like from the ssa.gov: Someone born on June 15,1946 could expect to live about 15-17 years longer.

Age	Additional Years of life expectancy	Estimated Total Years
Woman 70	16.7	87.7
Man 70	14.7	85.7

The government projects your Required Minimum Distribution (RMD) at age 70½.

The government RMD income could cause your accounts to be very depleted. Half of the people will live longer than projected. If you are lucky enough to be long lived, RMD's could deplete your account to almost nothing. RMD's will also increase the amount of taxes you owe.

There is a qualified longevity annuity contract (QLAC) that will protect some of your money from RMD's. QLACs provide some relief for about 15 years. At age 85 you will be required to begin taking the money out. Taxes will be required to be paid at that time. If you pass away, your estate and beneficiaries will pay the taxes.

Roth IRA withdrawals are non-taxed, and there is no RMD attached to Roth IRAs. Some people rollover their 401k into a Roth IRA. Taxes must be paid during the calendar year of the rollover. Doing this over several years may ease the financial pain, but ultimately, the government will get the taxes. You can leave money in a Roth, and it will not affect the taxes.

Withdrawal of money from the traditional IRA can be spread out over the expected lifetime of the primary heir. This will alleviate some of the tax burdens.

Consider what will happen to retirement monies when passed on to the beneficiaries. It can create a burden for them. For example, when a 401k account is passed to the beneficiary, the account must be emptied within the timeframe of nine months. All the money comes to the beneficiaries within one calendar year. This usually causes the rate for income taxes to go to the extreme high. A person may think they're leaving a lot of money to their children, but 25 percent to 40 percent of their account will go to the federal and state governments.

A Roth IRA left to your children, or other beneficiaries remain a tax-exempt income. The beneficiaries must empty the account eventually. The government enforces rules, so tax-free money does not go on for long periods.

The RMD income levels may cause an increase in Social Security taxes. There are significant negative financial consequences to leaving your money unprotected from RMD's.

You can avoid this if you plan for it. It requires you move your money. The best places to move your retirement money is to an annuity that will pay you a flat amount for a time period (10 years or more) or the rest of your life. Life insurance is a way to protect your money too.

You can turn a 401k into a tax-free account. It can be done relatively painlessly. Do it close to age 59 ½ to make it work the best. It requires an insurance account. Take the cash and buy a life insurance policy called indexed universal life. Add to the policy yearly with large amounts of money from the 401k. This is complicated, but greatly rewarding in the end.

INFLATION:
THE SILENT KILLER
OF FINANCES

CHAPTER 20

TERM LIFE INSURANCE

FINANCIAL ADVISORS ADVERTISE buying term life insurance instead of buying whole life insurance. Term life insurance is the most familiar and is always cheapest. When you have a young family, you get the most bang for your buck, from term life insurance. The advice is to buy term insurance and save or invest the money equal to a whole life policy payment. Hopefully, if you heeded this advice you invested "the rest." People have good intentions to invest the additional money, but they don't.

Employers may offer term life insurance as a benefit to employees. These term policies are usually cancelled at retirement or within a few years of retirement. Many people do not replace their company life insurance policy with a policy of their own. Reasons for not replacing the term policy are usually because of an increased cost or disqualification because of poor health.

Inaction with life insurance could be detrimental to your spouse. Most people want their spouse to have enough money to live life comfortably after they die.

Check your work term life insurance policy for a renewability clause. The clause allows the insured to renew the term policy on an annual basis. The primary drawback of keeping term insurance is the probable yearly increasing premiums as the policy is renewed. Eventually, it is expensive to pay the premium. But, if you are in poor health, at least you have a policy.

Some insurance policies have a clause to convert the term policy into a permanent one. Since you already own the policy, it will convert without a medical exam or medical history. The premiums are calculated at the age of conversion. Convert as soon as you retire.

Using an insurance strategy in retirement could get you a check for the rest of your life. The best approach is to purchase a single premium immediate annuity by converting other retirement accounts. Annuities are provided by insurance companies and are considered insurance products.

While other people will worry about their 401k, 403b, IRA or bank CD's lasting for as long as they live, you will be assured that you are getting a check every month for your lifetime.

Recap:

Convert your term life insurance into a whole life policy. It may get you a check for the rest of your life.

CHAPTER 21

WHOLE LIFE INSURANCE

WHOLE LIFE INSURANCE IS A PERMANENT life insurance policy and offers lifelong coverage. The premiums remain the same for as long as you live. Some policies have annual dividends. The death benefit is guaranteed.

When purchasing whole life, you will see the terms face value and cash value. These are completely two different accounts attached to the policy.

Face value is the dollar amount the beneficiary receives upon the passing of the insured. If you buy a $200,000.00 policy, that is the face value. If you die the day after the policy is activated, even if you only paid one premium payment, your beneficiary receives the $200,000.00 payout.

Cash value begins to build after the premiums have been paid over a period. When you pay premiums, part of it goes into the cash value. Good policy investment performance increases the policy cash value.

Whole life will pay about 5-6 percent interest or more on cash value. This is a better financial option than a CD at your local bank. If you had $50,000.00 in a paid-up whole life insurance policy, it would be growing every year. A paid-up policy will have a cash value that gains a guaranteed higher rate of interest than a CD.

You can take a loan from the policy, by borrowing against the cash value. Obtaining the loan is a painless and is usually a quick process. A credit check is not necessary to get a loan from life insurance. It must be paid back with interest. If you die before repaying, the amount will be subtracted from the loan money paid out.

A life insurance policy with a guaranteed rate of growth will pass on to your beneficiaries. When a life insurance policy has a named beneficiary, it bypasses probate court. Its money would not be subject to creditors. Life insurance money is income tax exempt.

Husbands, on average, die seven years before their wives. Often, the husband leaves his wife with a hospital bill, funeral costs and perhaps a nursing home bill. These costs can take up to half of the assets. Life insurance pays directly to the beneficiaries. Life insurance is exempt from these bills.

To repeat, life insurance is not subject to bill collectors. This includes hospitals, nursing homes, and state governments.

We tend to pay off our bills without understanding whether we are responsible for them. You are not accountable for the debts of the deceased. You do not need to use the life insurance money for these bills.

Life insurance is a safe way to grow money. Cash funds in life insurance grow faster than the rate of inflation.

Insurance accounts have guarantees, so the account will not lose money. It is a safe no risk, investment for seniors.

A whole life policy can be converted to paid-up policies. A paid-up policy does not require a monthly or annual premium.

A less expensive option for a permanent policy is called universal life. You can get a larger Insurance value such as $50,000.00 as compared to $15,000.00 for about the same amount of premium money.

After the age of 60, life insurance is easier to qualify for than long-term care insurance. This makes a whole life policy a good investment. A permanent life insurance policy usually has a level premium, meaning the premium will not increase year after year.

Indexed universal life, universal life, or whole life insurance does not expire. These permanent policies provide benefits for the insured such as the ability to easily borrow money paid into the policy, make available long-term care, and act as a type of tax-deferred savings account.

Recap:

Life insurance is a safe way to grow money.

AN AGING RETIREE

DOES NOT HAVE

TIME

TO RECOVER

FROM

STOCK MARKET LOSES

CHAPTER 23

LONG TERM CARE INSURANCE

LONG-TERM CARE INSURANCE is purchased to protect your estate from the cost of nursing homes or in-home care. This type of care is expensive. If Medicaid paid for these services, they would look for reimbursement from the estate.

Long term care insurance will protect the money in your estate from nursing homes, dollar for dollar. If the long-term care bills amount to more than your policy will pay, you or your estate will be responsible for up to half of those bills. This may vary from state to state.

Most states have a five-year look-back period for long-term care costs. This means there must be a plan for the dispersal of the estate more than five years before the needed in-home or nursing home care.

If you are not married and/or do not have a large estate, long-term care insurance will not make financial sense.

THINK AHEAD TO WHAT FINANCIAL FUTURE YOU WILL HAVE IF YOUR SPOUSE DIES

CHAPTER 24

FINAL EXPENSE INSURANCE

HOW MUCH DOES A FUNERAL cost? Transport of the body, embalming, visitation, wake, pastor, ceremony fees, burial, cemetery costs are the usual expenses for a funeral. Cremation will decrease the costs, but only minimally.

The average funeral runs between $7000.00-$8000.00. The cost includes the above services. A post funeral meal, music, speaker, or special venue are additional expenses to be considered. These payments can and do add up to even double the funeral costs.

Final expense insurance is a life policy that is flexible because you can purchase life insurance by one thousand-dollar increments. For example, you may anticipate that a funeral will cost about $15,000.00. The life policy can be written for this amount. Or if desired, a lesser amount like $7000.00 - $9,000.00 could be the amount that the policy pays out to the survivors.

Underwriting rules are not as strict for final expense insurance as compared to other permanent policies. People with medical conditions will be able to qualify for a policy. If you are already ill, it can be very expensive. The best time to buy it, of course, is when you don't need it.

Some people are reluctant to spend money on life insurance, especially when they are healthy. Death is unpredictable, couples should think ahead to what life would be like for a surviving spouse. The financial future of the survivor may be quite bleak. Upon death, many a spouse loses a third or more of the couple's income. If you lost a third of your income but got a chunk of money from life insurance, your life would be easier.

A funeral trust protects money from creditors. A funeral trust often pays more quickly than life insurance which can often take two weeks or more.

Have you considered donating your body to science? It saves you funeral money. It promotes medical learning for future doctors and scientists. It is helpful for research. This decision can be made before death or at the time of death. It is, however, easier if the deceased has made the decision.

Donating your body to science doesn't mean you forgo a funeral. You may still have a nice funeral ceremony but without the body. The deceased will go to a medical school or research facility for about three years. After that time, the research facility will pay for cremation and burial, essentially making the death expenses go away. Some families opt to have another ceremony at the burial.

No one wants loved ones to rack up credit card debt for their funeral. Get a dedicated funeral savings account, a final expense insurance or life policy. Help your family pay for your funeral expenses. They will thank you.

THE BEST TIME TO BUY

INSURANCE

IS

WHEN YOU DON'T NEED IT

It is important to plan for retirement. For the best health insurance coverage, you will need Medicare A, B, Supplement or Advantage plan and a drug plan.

Look at all your retirement funds. Move 401k and 403b and other taxable funds into safe annuity or insurance accounts.

Plan for life, illness and death. Plan for fun. Learn new skills, catch up on your favorite hobbies, volunteer, travel and enjoy your family. Turning 65 and entering retirement is a fantastic place to be!

If you do not have access to an agent, I am available for telephone or internet conferences. The consult is free. I will assist you to find the most appropriate plan for your situation. Licensure in your state is necessary to assist you.

I can recommend an agent in your area. As the owner of Retirement Planning Systems, my goal is to help people save and make money.

Contact information:

LYNN H. ZAFFKE

lzaffke@retirementplanningsystems.net

ISBN-13:
978-1548002978

ISBN-10:
1548002976

References

Hobbs, F., Damon, B., & Bernstein, R. (2011, October 31). SIXTY-FIVE PLUS IN THE UNITED STATES May 1995. Retrieved July 31, 2017, from https://www.census.gov/population/socdemo/statbriefs/agebrief.html

"Medicare & You 2016" Accessed August 08, 2016 https://www.medicare.gov/Pubs/pdf/10050.pdf

"Medicare & You 2017" Accessed May 25, 2017

Reliant Life Share Case Summary, Accessed May 25, 2017, http://reliantlifeshares.com/wp-content/uploads/2014/07/Reliant-Confidential-Investor-Policy-U00003278A.pdf

LIFE INSURANCE

HELPS

THE SURVIVORS

NOTES

NOTES

NOTES

www.ingramcontent.com/pod-product-compliance
Lightning Source LLC
Chambersburg PA
CBHW071216280526
45787CB00002B/705